Whole Food: The 30 Day Whole Food Diet Cookbook

The Best Recipes to Help You Lose Weight and Change Your Life!

FREE BONUSES

As Promised Here is Your 100 Diet Tips
CLICK HERE to Get Your Copy.

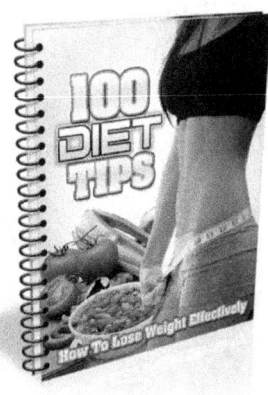

If You Want Free Best Selling Kindle Books Delivered To You Weekly CLICK HERE

TABLE OF CONTENTS

INTRODUCTION

I want to thank you and congratulate you for downloading the book, *Whole Food: The 30 Day Whole Food Diet Cookbook* This book contains proven steps and strategies on how to live a healthier and happier life while on the whole food guide.

The whole food diet is an amazing program that has helped me and countless others on it. It helps you feel healthier and more refreshed than ever before. The book lists some of the benefits that you will see while on the diet and has some tips and tricks to help you stay on the diet. As you read on, we will challenge some of the misconceptions associated with the diet and inform you about facts that you never knew! This really is a delightful diet to be on and I hope that you benefit from it as much as we have.

Thanks again for downloading this book, I hope you enjoy it!

CHAPTER 1

What is a Whole Food Diet?

Anyone who is even reasonably interested in their nutrition and diet must have come across the term 'Whole Foods' at some point or another. It is a dietary preference that is becoming increasingly popular with dieticians and nutritionists all over the world. A large number of celebrities including Josh Duhamel and Chris Hemsworth have recently come on board the diet plan and are religiously following it. But, what exactly are whole foods and what can they do for you? These are the common questions that we come across every day and hope to answer with this e-book. Although the term is widely known, few people know what it consists of and how easy it is to incorporate it as a part of your daily life.

A whole-food diet is essentially a diet that consists of eating food in its purest form. It is based on a true 'farm to table' concept that has gained so much popularity in the recent years. Unlike the common misconception, it does not involve actually eating your food in full. Nor, does it involve food bought only from 'Whole Foods', the organic grocery giant. Although, the philosophy of the company is quite similar, both concentrating on organic and fresh produce. A whole food diet consists of eating fresh fruits, vegetables, and grains which have been subjected to minimal outside influence. The food that you eat in this diet is made from ingredients that are almost as pure as they would occur in nature.

The philosophy behind a whole-foods diet is that if it was good enough for our ancestors, then it is good enough for us. The use of Pesticides, plant food, and other chemicals are mostly a recent invention. Preserved and pre-packed meals, also take away a lot of nutrition from our meals. These methods take away the nutrient value of the food by such a huge amount, that we get only a fraction of the benefit from it that we should be getting. Whole foods consist of fresh produce like fruits, vegetables, grains, beans, and legumes which are consumed in their natural form. The diet seeks to minimize meat intake and processed foods as much as possible by reducing or eliminating them from the diet. Even additives like salt, fats and preservatives are prohibited in this diet. Dairy is the only thing that is considered better consumed after processing as the process does not drastically alter the nutrient value and also unpasteurized milk and milk products can cause severe illnesses.

CHAPTER 2

The Difference between Organic and Whole Foods

A common confusion between health enthusiasts is regarding the exact difference between whole foods and Organic produce, both of which have a wide following. Simply put, while a lot of organic foods are considered whole foods, it is not necessary that all whole foods are organic in nature.

Organic food consists of produce in which modern farming technologies like pesticides, irradiation, and bio-engineering practices have not been applied. They are free from chemicals and antibiotics, and thus considered healthier to eat. Whole foods consist of food made from unprocessed ingredients which can include fruits, vegetables, dairy. and grains. They are free from any additives and preservative and thus as close to those occurring in nature as possible. Organic food can very successfully be assimilated to a whole foods diet as they are considered both ethical farming and have proven to be healthier and more nutritional. It is recommended to add organic produce to your Whole foods diet to make it even more beneficial for you.

Organic farming is considered an ethical practice as the food grown by this method does not harm nature as much as non-organic items. The produce limit's the environmental damage by not using pesticides and fertilizer which are disposed into water bodies and thus harm their natural habitats. Whole food has little to do with environmental benefit but is more of a personal dietary preference. It's concentration in on providing a healthy meal on the table rather than protecting the environment. However, there is no harm in using organic produce for a whole food diet. By incorporating both these things in your diet, you can live both a healthier and greener lifestyle.

CHAPTER 3

Benefits of Whole Foods

A whole foods diet can cause tremendous changes in your lifestyle from Day 1. When eating fresh food every day becomes a part of your routine, you not only feel much healthier but start to see the benefits of going on the diet. Some of the many advantages of switching to a whole food diet are listed below:

Although weight loss is not one of the main objectives of a whole food diet, it is a benefit that comes naturally along with a whole food diet. A lot of fatty food items like processed meat and pre-packaged food are naturally eliminated from this diet. This reduces the calorie intake drastically and also the food you consume in this diet is much easier for the body to metabolize. But this does not mean that you are not getting the nutrition that you need! In fact, a whole food diet stresses on consuming the necessary calorie intake according to your body type but eliminating all that is excess. This means that if you were living an unhealthy lifestyle earlier, you loose a lot of weight without having to ever stay hungry!

Going on a whole food diet has a variety of health benefits. It is especially recommended for people who have high blood sugar, high blood pressure, and digestion problems. This diet eliminates processed sugar and includes a lot of naturally occurring protein sources. Plant-based proteins do a much better job of controlling your blood sugar levels than animal based ones. Also, most of the ingredients are rich in fiber and are eaten in the form that makes it easy for the body to digest the food. Another health Benefit that has been seen is that people on this diet have been known to experience considerably less muscle pain. Food items rich in animal fat have been known to increase inflammation in muscles and joints. The high acidic content of this food makes it hard for the body to recover naturally. While, a green, nutritious and fibrous whole food promotes healing when muscle pain occurs.

Our bodies have been made in a way in which it finds it much easier to break down food that occurs naturally. Before modern technology, human beings have naturally been eating whole foods for thousands of years and have lived happy and healthy lives. Since whole foods are easier to digest, they put considerably less stress on the body. This results in higher energy levels for you. Whole foods when eaten correctly contain all the carbohydrates, plant protein, fiber, and fat that your body needs to stay healthy and energetic.

Once you start on a whole food diet, you will find it impossible to go back to your old eating habits. Fresh and Natural foods are much tastier and delicious than processed food. The variety of recipes and meal plans that you can experiment with are endless. Our taste buds have been set by Mother Nature herself to appreciate fresh fruits and vegetables. In fact, a lot of them are delicious even when eaten raw, without the help of any spices and cooking. There is no meat product that you can consume without having to cook it properly. Who would want to go back to eating packaged food items after eating food fresh from the garden?

CHAPTER 4

Whole Food: A 30 Day Whole Food Challenge

A 30-day whole food diet is a great option for those looking to live the whole food lifestyle. It only takes as little as 30 days to see the difference in your weight and overall health once you start on the diet. The chapters ahead contain some delicious recipes that break the myth that a mostly vegetarian diet cannot be as tasty. We have prepared recipes according to Breakfast, lunch, Dinner and Snack time which you can mix and match according to your mood and what is in your refrigerator. The only thing that you need to keep in mind is that the ingredients that you are using. There is no need to spend hours calorie counting when you are on the whole food diet because the recipes are filling and naturally low in calories. As long as you do not go overboard and limit the quantities of certain high-calorie ingredients, you are good to go! We are sure that once you take up the 30-day challenge, you will never go back to your old diet!

To help you stay on track, here are some ingredients that you can and cannot have while on the diet.

Do's: Fresh Fruits, Fresh Vegetables, Unprocessed grains like Beans and Legumes, Dairy products like fresh milk and homemade yogurt, nuts, seeds. Anything that does not have any additives or preservatives and has not been processed in any way at all is allowed on this diet.

Don't: Processed and packaged food items, 'Junk' food of any sort, Soda, Alcohol, Tobacco, Processed sugar, anything containing MSG or sulfites. Meat products should be avoided or kept to a minimum.

CHAPTER 5

BASICS

This section contains some recipes that you will see frequently in this cookbook. Most of us consider whole foods limiting, due to the unavailability of certain ingredients without additives or preservatives. You can easily prepare these ingredients and sauces before hand and store them in the refrigerator for at least a week, even some longer. Preparing these are not only easy on the pockets, but you will also see the difference in the taste in the food that you prepare.

Homemade Chili Sauce

Preparation Time: 15 minutes

Cooking Time: 10 minutes

Makes: 1 Bowl

2 tsp Chili Powder

1 Tomato

3 cloves crushed garlic

½ tsp salt

2 Dried red chili

Step 1: Boil the tomatoes and peel them once they cool off. The skins should come off on their own boiled once. Blend into a smooth puree for about 1 minute and strain to thin it out.

Step 2: Place the chili powder, dried red chili, crushed garlic, salt, and the tomato puree into the blender and blend until a smooth sauce.

Step3: Refrigerate for about a week and use as needed.

Homemade Cream

Preparation Time: 60 mins (not taking into account the collecting time)

Cooking Time: 10 mins

Portions: 1 Bowl

Ingredients:

Milk

Step 1: This recipe is meant to be made over time and is not a one-time process. You can collect the cream every time you boil milk. Every time before you use milk for something, boil it in a large pot for about 5 minutes and let it cool.

Step 2: After around an hour of cooling, you will be able to see a thick layer of cream on top. Use a spoon to take out the cream and store it in a container. You can use the milk as you would use it normally. You can collect as much cream as you want, depending on how frequently you boil your milk.

Step 3: Keep collecting cream for about 10 days and storing it in the same airtight container. Once you have enough cream, place all the cream in a blender and blend it until it is smooth.

Step 4: Refrigerate the cream in an airtight container and use as needed. This cream is an unsweetened cream and supposed to be used for gravies, soups and savories only. Please do not use it for dessert as the sour taste is not suitable for it.

Homemade Butter

Preparation Time: 10 mins

Cooking Time: None

Ingredients:

2 cups Homemade cream (prepared as above)

½ tsp Salt (optional)

1 cup Water

Step 1: Place all the ingredients into a blender and blend for about 10-15 minutes. The butter should separate by the time you are done.

Step 2: Strain off the excess water and add salt according to taste. Refrigerate and use as needed.

Homemade Yogurt

Preparation Time: 6-8 hours for setting the curd

Cooking Time: 10 mins

Ingredients:

500 ml of Full-Fat Milk

1 tbsp curd.

Step 1: Heat the milk in a large pot for about 10-15 minutes on medium heat. Bring the milk to a boil until a creamy layer forms on top. Take it off the stove.

Step 2: Cool down the milk till it is lukewarm and add a tbsp of curd. Mix the curd well until it dissolves completely.

Step 3: Cover and cool the milk-curd mixture for about 6-8 hours until it sets completely.

Homemade Sour Cream

Preparation Time: 5 mins

Cooking Time: None

Ingredients:

1 cup fresh cream

2 tbsp Homemade Yogurt

2 tsp Lemon juice

Salt to taste

Ingredients:

Step 1: Take a large bowl and mix all the above ingredients. Whisk well until it is completely smooth.

Step 2: Cool it in a refrigerator for about 4 hours until it thickens. Use it as needed for about a week.

Homemade Cottage Cheese

Preparation Time: 30 mins

Cooking Time: 5 mins

Portions: 1 Block

Ingredients:

1 ltr Full-fat Milk

2 tbsp lemon juice

Step 1: Place the milk in a large pot and bring to a boil. Add the lemon juice once the milk starts to boil. The milk will start to curdle.

Step 2: Remove it from the stove when the milk starts to curdle. Strain the milk using a cheesecloth to drain the whey.

Step 3: Tie the cheesecloth tightly so that the milk shred are pulled tightly together.

Step 4: Place the cloth on a plate and place some weight on top of the cloth.

Step 5: In about 30-40 minutes, the cottage cheese should have set. Put the cottage cheese block in an air-tight container filled with water. Store it in a refrigerator and use as needed for about 5 days.

Homemade Vegetable Stock

Preparation Time: 15 mins

Cooking Time: 30 mins

Portions: 1 Ltr

Ingredients:

1 onion

2 Celery Stalks

2 carrots

1 bunch Green Onions

8 Chopped Garlic Cloves

1 tbsp chopped parsley

1 tbsp chopped thyme

2-3 Bay Leaves

1 tsp Salt

Step 1: Wash all the vegetables thoroughly to remove the soil. Chop all the vegetables into large chunks.

Step 2: Heat the oil in a large pot. Lightly saute the onion, garlic, parsley, thyme, and celery for about 5 mins.

Step 3: Add around 4 cups of water to the same pot where the herbs are getting cooked. Add all the vegetables to the pot. Let it cook on low heat for about half an hour so that the water is infused with the flavors of the vegetables. Cover the pot while it is getting cooked. You can use almost any vegetable scraps to prepare this broth, including stems, leaves, skins, and roots of vegetables. You can also choose to add veggies like mushrooms, asparagus, and eggplant which will give out the flavor but not melt completely in the broth.

Step 4: Strain the water and discard the vegetables and herbs. Store the stock in an airtight bottle and refrigerate. Use it as need for 10-15 days.

Homemade Tomato Puree

Preparation Time: 10 mins

Cooking Time: 10 mins

Portions: 1 Bowl

Ingredients:

4 Tomatoes

Salt to taste

Step 1: Boil the tomatoes in a large pot full of water. The peels will start coming off naturally once the tomatoes are boiled.

Step 2: Drain the tomatoes and let it cool. Peel off any skin that has not already come off. Scoop out as much seed as possible and cut into large chunks.

Step 3: Blend the puree in a blender until there are no lumps and the puree is smooth. Drain the puree using a sieve or use as it is. Refrigerate in an airtight container and use as required.

CHAPTER 6

BREAKFAST RECIPES

E verybody has heard since childhood that a breakfast is the most important meal of the day. It is a simple fact which everybody knows but few take into consideration in their daily lives. A healthy breakfast has the incredible potential to jumpstart your day with energy and enthusiasm. Your body naturally burns out the calories you consume during the beginning of the day because of the activities that lie ahead. But, it is much harder to burn those calories which are consumed later in the day. So, even in terms of weight loss, one should take the advantage of consuming a filling meal in the morning so that they feel less hungry throughout the day. Here are some healthy and nutritious recipes that are sure to bring a smile to your face in the morning.

A Whole Breakfast Burrito

A breakfast burrito is the favorite breakfast-on-the-go for many people. A lot of people cannot even imagine getting to have one while on a diet. But, a whole food version of a breakfast burrito is not just a healthy but also a filling breakfast option. Grated potatoes are used to create the 'Dough' for the burrito and topped with succulent, gorgeous veggies and 'cheesy' yeast.

Prep Time: 30 mins

Cooking Time: 60 mins

Portions: 8

Ingredients:

3 Peeled Potatoes

3 Tbsp Yeast

½ Onion, Diced

1 Bell Pepper of your choice, Diced

10 small Portobello mushrooms, Sliced

1 bunch of chopped Spinach

Lime Juice

2 tbsp chopped basil

2 cloves chopped garlic

1 ½ Tsp chopped Oregano

1 tsp Chili Powder

½ tsp chili flakes

1 cup Diced Tomatoes

1 Cups Boiled Black Beans

1 Cup boiled Pinto Beans

2 Tbsp Chopped Cilantro

Step 1: Shred the potatoes using a shredder while they are still raw. Fill up an open pressure cooker or a large soup pot with around an inch of water. Use a steamer basket to steam the shredded potatoes. Make sure that the water is below the basket and does not overflow onto the potatoes. Once the potatoes are soft, take them out of the steamer and divide them into 2 equal parts. Add about 2 tbsp of yeast to one portion of the shredded potatoes.

Step 2: In a separate pan, saute the garlic, onions and bell peppers with a little bit of water in that order. The water should be used in a small quantity just so that the veggies do not stick to the pan. After the veggies are cooked in about 3-4 minutes, add the spinach. After around 2 minutes, add 2 tbsp of lime juice, oregano, basil, chili powder and chili flakes. Add 1 tbsp of yeast and the potatoes without the yeast. Lower the heat and add the beans, tomatoes, and garnish with cilantro leaves.

Step 3: Spread the mixture evenly over a small rectangular baking dish. Spread the potatoes with the yeast in another even layer over the layer of veggies. Bake this at around 375 degrees for 35 minutes. Check if the top layer has browned. If not, then bake for another 10 minutes. Serve while still hot for a delicious breakfast.

Cauliflower Hash Browns

Cauliflowers are some of the most versatile vegetables that exist. They take on the flavor of almost any dish that they are put into and acquire a tremendous taste that is both distinctive and delicious. Although the traditional hash browns can also be a part of the whole food diet, a cauliflower hash brown is a much less fatty and much more healthy alternative for those looking to lose some weight. The best part is that this delicious dish can be prepared at a moments notice, requires very few ingredients, and fills you up for a long part of the day.

Prep Time: 5-10 mins

Cooking Time: 10 mins

Portions: 2

Ingredients:

Olive Oil

½ Cauliflower floret chopped finely

1 Diced Onion

1 tbsp Chopped Garlic

2 tbsp Lemon Juice

2 tsp chopped Parsley

1 tsp Chili Flakes

¼ tsp black pepper

Salt to Taste

Step 1: Mix the cauliflowers and onions in a bowl. Heat about 2 tbsp of olive oil on a large pan/ skillet. You can also use water if you do not want to include oil in your diet, but a little bit of oil is fine. Once the oil heats up, spread the cauliflower-onion mixture on the skillet as an even layer. Do not stir or sauté the mixture and let it take a shape as it gets cooked for about 2 minutes.

Step 2: Add the chili flakes, salt, pepper, and around 2 tbsp of water. Stir and mix the mixture and spread it evenly again. Cover and cook until the water is cooked for about 5 mins maximum. Check and make sure that the cauliflower is cooked by piercing it with a fork. The mixture should have a golden color.

Step 3: Reduce the heat and add the chopped garlic. Cook for another 2 mins while stirring continuously. Once this is cooked, add the lemon juice to the mixture and stir.

Step 4: Plate up the scrambled cauliflower and garnish with freshly chopped parsley.

Scrambled Potatoes

Scrambled Potatoes are a mouth-watering substitute for scrambled eggs and taste heavenly with toast. It is just a wholesome, comfort food filled with juicy vegetables and goodness. It is slightly higher in calorie content than the other dishes but breakfast is supposed to be ideally the most filling meal of the day. You can compensate with a lighter lunch and dinner to see effective results. This scrambled potatoes recipe is sure to give you enough energy for your whole day.

Prep Time: 30 mins

Cooking Time: 40 mins

Portions: 5

Ingredients:

4 Medium Potatoes

1 Chopped Onion

1/3 Chopped Red Bell Pepper

1/3 Chopped Yellow Bell Pepper

1/3 Chopped Green Red Pepper

4 Sliced Mushrooms

1 tsp Chopped Oregano

1 tsp Chopped Basil

1 tsp Red Chili Flakes

1 cup cooked white beans

1 chopped tomato

A few chopped Spinach leaves

Optional: Homemade Salsa For Topping (recipe below)

Step 1: Chop the raw potatoes into bite-sized cubes without taking the skin off. Spread the cubes onto a baking sheet and place it in an over preheated to about 375 degrees. Flip the potatoes after about 15 minutes of baking so that the potatoes are crispy and evenly cooked. Bake for another 15 minutes and keep them aside.

Step 2 (Optional): Chop tomatoes, onions, basil, garlic, green peppers, and cilantro into as small pieces as possible. Mix it all in a bowl and add red chili powder, salt, pepper, and lime juice to taste. Store in the fridge and serve chilled.

Step 3: Take a large pan or skillet and heat a tbsp of water or oil as per your dietary preference. Add the onions and saute for a while. After about a minute, add the bell peppers and the mushrooms. Cook for about 2-3 mins until the vegetables are soft and colorful and the water is absorbed. Add the chopped garlic and stir for a bit. Then add the chopped herbs like oregano, basil and chili flakes.

Step 4: Reduce the heat and add the white beans, spinach, and chopped tomatoes. The tomatoes and spinach should give out water naturally but add more water or stock if the food starts to stick. Once the water is almost evaporated, mix in the potatoes and top with the salsa and serve.

Whole Oat Muffins

Oatmeal and bran are two grains that are both permissible in a whole food diet and easily adaptable to a variety of breakfast recipes. The amazing thing about the muffins is they taste equally great when sweetened or unsweetened. Muffins are an excellent go-to breakfast which you can cook in advance, store in your refrigerator and just grab on the way to work or school. The healthy grains in this muffin also makes it much lower in calories than the store-bought version.

Prep Time: 10-15 mins

Cooking Time: 15 mins

Portions: 12 Muffins

Ingredients:

2.5 Cups of Oats-Bran

2 tsp Baking Powder (Recipe Below)

1.5 tsp Salt adjusted to taste

2 tsp Cinnamon

2 Eggs (optional)

2/3 Cup Vegetable Glycerin

2 Tsp Vanilla Extract

4 tsp Clarified Butter or Ghee

A few almonds

Step 1: Baking Powder Substitute: Blend a 2 tbsp of Baking Soda, 4 tbsp of tartar cream, and 3 tbsp of cornstarch. Blend all the ingredients thoroughly. Store in an air-tight container and use as a substitute for baking powder.

Step 2: Mix the oat bran, baking powder, salt, cinnamon powder, and nuts in a bowl.

Step 3: Mix the egg whites and yolk, vegetable glycerin, ghee, and vanilla with around ¾ cup of water until no lumps are left.

Step 4: Grease the muffin trays with clarified butter/ghee and preheat the oven to around 400 degrees.

Step 5: Put the dish in once the oven is heated and bake for around 15-20 minutes. Keep checking after 10 minutes are over if the center of the muffins has set. Remove from the tray once it cools down and enjoy!

You can easily prepare a non-sweetened, savory version of this muffin by eliminating the cinnamon, vegetable glycerin, and vanilla extract. The rest of the recipe remains as it is.

Whole Waffles

Whole waffles made from delicious oatmeal and topped with strawberry syrup are just as delicious as the regular ones. An earthy, grainy texture, topped with fresh fruits and honey makes for an excellent start to your day. Serve it to someone on a processed food diet and we are sure that they will be able to barely tell the difference, if at all.

Prep Time: 20 mins

Cooking Time: 5 mins

Portions: 6 Classic Waffles

Ingredients:

3 cups of milk

¼ cup raw cashew nuts, without the skin

2 tbsp clarified butter/ghee

1.5 cups of grounded oats

½ cup of cornmeal

2 tsp baking powder (or substitute as given in the previous recipe)

½ tsp cinnamon powder

An assortment of berries for toppings, chopped

1 cup pureed strawberry, mixed with ½ tsp sugar

Step 1: Mix the butter and 2 cups of milk in a bowl and blend it until it is smooth and there are no lumps. Keep it aside while you prepare the other ingredients.

Step 2: Mix the oatmeal and cornmeal in a bowl. Add the baking and cinnamon powder to the mixture and mix thoroughly. Grease your waffle iron with the clarified butter so that the waffle does not stick and Heat your waffle iron up to the medium setting.

Step 3: Mix the milk mixture into the oats mixture and whisk until no lumps exist. Let the mixture rest for a few minutes and add a few tbsp of milk if needed before cooking if the batter thickens too much.

Step 4: If you are making classic waffles, pour around a ½ cup of the batter onto your stove and close the lid for around 3 minutes until the indicators start to beep or blink. If you are making Belgian waffles, the process should take around 5 mins and require around 1 cup of batter for each waffle.

Step 5: Serve hot. Top it with your choice of sliced berries and a delicious drizzle of honey and pureed strawberries.

Breakfast Smoothie

A breakfast smoothie is the perfect quickie option for a breakfast. You can just take any of the healthy fruits and veggies from your refrigerator, blend them in one quick motion with some yogurt and have a breakfast ready within minutes! A smoothie naturally needs less sugar but you can try substituting the sugar with fresh honey for a much healthier option. This is an amazing breakfast option for those hot, summer days when you just don't feel like having anything warm or heavy in the morning. As an added bonus, a smoothie is also incredibly easy and you can easily teach almost anybody, including your kids how to make it!

Prep Time: 10 mins

Cook Time: None!

Blend Time: 2-3 mins

Serves: 2

Ingredients:

A cup full of your favorite fresh fruits chopped into large pieces.

1 Glass Milk

½ cup yogurt

Sugar/ Honey to taste

Step 1: Throw in all the ingredients in a blender and blend until smooth. Check the consistency of the smoothie and add water or milk as needed. Taste and add the sugar/ honey according to preference. Serve chilled.

CHAPTER 7

LUNCH RECIPES

A lot of people make the mistake of rushing through their breakfast with a light meal and then indulging in fatty and high-calorie foods during the lunch hours. One way to avoid those lunchtime hunger pangs is to have a nutritious and filling breakfast which gets naturally digested because of all the day's work and treating you to a lighter and healthier lunch. Soups, salads, and sandwiches make ideal lunch options as they are quick to make, easy to carry, and light to eat. Here are some lunch recipes that are guaranteed to brighten up your day and get rid of those lunch-time cravings while you are on the Whole Food Diet.

Hearty Vegetable Soup

This wholesome vegetable soup is filled with the goodness of all the vegetables that you can get from your garden. It is a colorful and flavorful mélange of the most beautiful veggies that you can think of. The best thing about it is that you can do your prep while you cook by just adding the veggies to the pot as you chop them which cuts your cooking time into half of what I have written here. You can easily modify this recipe to suit your favorite vegetables and herbs. Just make sure that you have at least 3-4 veggies so that you get a flavor in the broth. It tastes delicious no matter what vegetable you choose to add to it.

Prep Time: 15 mins

Cooking Time: 25 mins

Serves: 4 Portions

Ingredients:

1 Peeled Potato

1 Onion Diced

1-2 Carrots Diced

1 Cup Green Beans

1 cup Broccoli Florets

2 Tbsp Pureed Tomatoes

1 tsp Chopped Garlic

A Dash of Olive Oil

2 Tbsp Chopped Parsley

1 Stick of Celery

½ tsp dried oregano

salt and pepper to taste

Step 1: Take a large pot with 5-6 cups of water and put it to a boil.

Step 2: In a separate pan, sauté the garlic with just a small dash of olive oil.

Step 3: Add the potatoes to the water once it starts to boil. Next, chop the celery and then add them to the broth. The celery is what gives the aroma to the stock so make sure to add it to the beginning.

Step 4: Next just keep adding the other vegetables as you chop them to the pot. Start with the ones which take the longest to cook and end with the ones that cook the fastest. Add the onions, carrots, beans, and broccoli in that order. Let it cook for 15-20 minutes over medium heat until all the vegetables are cooked.

Step 5: Once the vegetables are soft, add the sautéed garlic to the pot along with the oil if there is any left. Next, add the tomato puree, dried oregano, and the chopped herbs. Add salt and freshly ground black pepper to taste.

Step 6: Remove and serve hot with a side of whole wheat bread and garden salad.

Carrot, Tomato and Bell Pepper Soup

Would you believe that a luscious, creamy tomato soup like this one needs no cream at all! And yet it is true. Made with whole tomatoes, bell peppers and little else, this soup is as nutritious as it is tasty. The best part is that you never even feel like there is anything missing. This soup also looks gorgeous on the table if you are expecting guests over. A beautiful red color and mouth-watering taste, what more could you ask for?

Prep Time: 10 mins

Cook Time: 20 mins

Portions: 4 cups

Ingredients:

2-3 Tomatoes

1 Bell Pepper, diced

1 Carrot, diced

1 tsp Homemade Butter

1 tsp chopped basil

Salt and Pepper to taste

Step 1: Take a large pot and fill it halfway with water. Once the water heats up, add the whole tomatoes, carrots, and bell pepper until the vegetables are boiled. You can add a pinch of salt to speed up the boiling process. The tomatoes will boil fairly fast and start to peel off on its own once done.

Step 2: Once all the vegetables are tender, drain out the water through a sieve. Peel the tomatoes and wait for the vegetable to cool down.

Step 3: Chop the tomatoes into large chunks once they have cooled down. Then, put all three vegetables into a mixer/grinder, blender or food processor, along with a little bit of water and blend it until they become a smooth puree. Check and see if there are any lumps and blend it once more if needed.

Step 4: Filter the pureed tomato, bell pepper, and carrot mixture through a large sieve. This will help your soup get the creamy texture that we are looking for.

Step 5: Heat the puree in a large pot over medium heat. Add water if consistency is very thick. Add the homemade butter and basil to the puree. Heat it till it comes to a boil. Then add salt and freshly ground black pepper according to taste. Serve hot with a side of garden salad.

Roasted Squash Soup

Once you get the hang of the basic idea, you can easily use any combination of vegetables to make a soup using the same method. A roasted squash soup is not a soup that requires a lot of innovation, but is a great soup, all the same. It is heavy enough to be had for dinner and is a delicious winter-time soup for those cold months when all you need is a hearty soup to make you feel all warm inside.

Prep Time: 5 mins

Cooking Time: 20 mins

Portions: 4 cups

Ingredients:

1 Mid-sized Butternut Squash

1 Sweet Potato

2 Bowls homemade Vegetable Stock (recipe in Basics)

2 Tbsp Lime Juice

Salt and Freshly Ground Black Pepper to taste

Step 1: Preheat your oven to around 400 degrees.

Step 2: While the oven heats up, cut your squash into large chunks and make sure to remove the seeds from it. Take your sweet potato and pierce it using a fork or knife in a few places. This will speed up the roasting and make sure that it is cooked evenly.

Step 3: Place all the vegetables on a baking sheet and spread them so that they are cooked evenly. Cook them for about an hour, turning them every 20 minutes.

Step 4: Remove them from the baking sheet after and hour. The vegetables should be soft and mushy. Peel the potatoes and squash and wait for them to cool a little bit.

Step 5: Place all the cooked vegetables in a blender/food processor. Add around 2 cups of vegetable broth to it and blend for around a minute until it becomes a smooth puree.

Step 6: Transfer the puree to a pot and bring to a boil. Add salt and pepper according to your taste. I use approximately half a teaspoon of each. Add the lemon juice to it for a hint of tangy flavor.

Step 7: Serve hot with a side of garden salad.

Asian Coleslaw

Do not be fooled into thinking that this is a traditional coleslaw salad. I am sure we are all bored of that one. This salad made from Asian purple Cabbage uses much of the same ingredients but is much more suitable as a lunchbox meal option if you are looking for a light lunch. If you are accustomed to heavier lunches. You can also spread it on whole wheat bread to make a tasty sandwich.

Preparation Time: 20 mins

Cooking Time: 5 mins

Portions: 2

Ingredients:

½ a Purple Cabbage(Should chop into approximately 4 cups)

1 Shredded Carrot

2 Thinly Sliced Radishes

1 Large Boiled Potato, Diced

3 tbsp Chopped Mint Leaves

2 Tbsp Toasted Sesame Seeds

½ tbsp olive oil

2 tbsp lemon juice

½ tbsp homemade chili sauce (Recipe in Basics)

½ tbsp Honey

2 tbsp Chopped Cilantro

Salt to taste

Step 1: Lightly toast the sesame seeds in a frying pan for approximately one minute until it turns a light, golden color.

Step 2: Place all the vegetables like the cabbage, potatoes, carrots, radishes, and the mint leaves in a large salad bowl.

Step 3: Prepare the dressing separately. Place the olive oil, lemon juice, homemade chili sauce, honey, salt and chopped cilantro together in a blender to make the dressing. Blend until smooth and creamy. Add a few tbsp of water if the consistency is too thick.

Step 4: Drizzle around 2-3 tbsp of dressing on the mixed vegetables. Mix to make sure the dressing is distributed evenly. Garnish with the toasted sesame seeds and serve with some extra dressing on the side.

Wild Rice, Spinach, and Beet Salad

The three key ingredients in this recipe combine to give you a gorgeous diversity in your plate. All three are so distinctive in terms of color and taste, yet they go amazingly well with each other. I have written this recipe as a salad but heated up it tastes equally good as a stir fry rice dish. The reds, greens, and browns come together and looks so beautiful on your plate that you are sure that it is delicious even before your first bite.

Preparation Time: 20 mins

Cooking Time: 30 mins

Portions: 4 bowls

Ingredients:

2 bunches of Chopped Spinach leaves

1 Cup wild rice, soaked for about 15 minutes

2 Cups Boiled and Diced Beets

1 Cup white beans (pre-soaked for at least 8 hours)

2 tbsp finely chopped garlic

3 Tbsp Sesame Oil

2 Tbsp Rice Wine Vinegar

2 Tbsp Soy Sauce

¼ cup freshly squeezed lemon juice

Salt and Sugar to taste

Step 1: Boil the rice, beets, and the beans in separate utensils as all three have different cooking times. The rice should be just slightly undercooked as this adds to the texture of the salad. Let them cool for a while if serving as a salad. You can also do this step on a weekend and store them in the refrigerator.

Step 2: In a large pan, lightly sauté the garlic for about a minute in about a tbsp of sesame oil until tender. If you are serving it as a warm salad or a stir fry, add the spinach leaves and cook them for about 30 seconds too.

Step 3: In a small bowl, prepare the salad dressing. Add the sesame oil, soy sauce, vinegar, lemon juice, and salt to taste. Add a pinch of sugar if needed, depending on your taste preference. Mix all the ingredients well and keep aside.

Step 4: In a large salad bowl, mix the rice, beets, beans, sautéed garlic and the spinach leaves. Drizzle a few tbsp of dressing on top of the salad and serve the balance dressing on the side.

Brown Rice Stir-Fry

Brown rice is an ingredient commonly used in whole food diets as a substitute for rice. It is much healthier and has a marginally less calorie content than regular rice. It has a delicious, chewy texture with almost a risotto like taste to it. It also contains a generous helping of nutrients like protein, fibers, and selenium. Brown rice, when combined with veggies makes for a beautiful plate that is a riot of colors. Here is a recipe that is quick to make and a great one for those lunch boxes.

Prep Time: 15 mins

Cooking Time: 20 mins

Portions: Four Bowls

Ingredients:

2 cups Brown Rice

2 tbsp clarified butter/ ghee

1 tbsp chopped garlic

½ cup chopped onions

1 cup chopped assorted bell peppers

½ cup chopped tomatoes

½ tsp dried oregano

½ tbsp chopped parsley

1 tsp chili powder

Salt and Pepper to taste

Step 1: Take a large pot with around 4 cups of water and heat it. Once the water is warm, add the rice to it and let it boil for about 15 minutes until tender. Drain the rice and wash it with cold water so that the grains do not stick together. Keep it aside and let it drain out while you prepare the vegetables.

Step 2: Take a large skillet and heat a tbsp of oil in it. Add the chopped garlic and sauté it for about a minute on medium heat until the garlic takes a light gold color. Next, add the onions and saute for about a minute until the onions become slightly translucent. Then, add the bell peppers and cook for a while. Add a pinch of salt to speed up the cooking process.

Step 3: Once the vegetables are cooked, add the chopped tomatoes and herbs. Let the tomatoes give out the water and get soft. Mash the tomatoes so that they become like a chunky gravy. Add the salt, pepper, and chili powder and cook for a minute.

Step 4: Add the drained and cooked rice to the vegetable mixture. Mix thoroughly so that the rice absorbs the tomato gravy properly. Garnish with chopped parsley and serve hot.

Yummy Chickpea Salad

Chickpeas are a great legume for those on the whole foods diet because they have an incredible taste, high in protein and give you the energy you need to keep raring to go all day. In fact, research shows that it can actually help reduce blood cholesterol! When combined with some yummy veggies, as in this salad, it makes a mouth-watering lunch that is easy to carry and quick to make! You only have to make sure that you soak the chickpeas overnight and then boil and keep them in the refrigerator. You can easily store boiled chickpeas for around a week and there are so many things that you can do with them, that you are sure to use them all before they go bad.

Prep Time: 20 mins

Cooking Time: None!

Serves: 4

Ingredients:

2 Cups Boiled Chickpeas

1 Cucumber, Chopped

1 Tomato, Chopped

1 Medium White Onion, Chopped

2 Tbsp Cilantro, Chopped

¼ cup Fresh Lemon Juice

Salt and Pepper to taste

Step 1: Toss all the ingredients together and serve chilled! Adjust the salt, pepper, and lemon juice according to taste.

HEALTHY VEGGIE BURGER

Preparation Time: 30 mins

Cooking Time: 40 mins

Portions: 4 Burgers

Ingredients:

4 whole wheat buns

2 Large Boiled potatoes

1 bowl boiled and finely chopped beans and carrots

1 Tomato Sliced

1 Onion Sliced

4 tbsp olive oil

2 tbsp tomato puree

2 tbsp Sour Cream (recipe in Basics)

¼ cup homemade chili sauce

A few Leaves of Iceberg Lettuce

1 tsp freshly ground chili powder

Salt and Pepper to taste

Step 1: Peel the boiled potatoes and mash them until there are no lumps. Finely chop the boiled beans and carrots and add them to the mashed potatoes. Add the chili powder and salt to taste. Mash them all together.

Step 2: Distribute the mashed potatoes into 4 sections and roll them into a smooth, round patty. Try to avoid any breaks in the patty. Place in the refrigerator for around 20 mins so that it becomes firmer.

Step 3: Heat up 2 tbsp of oil in a large frying pan. Place the patties on the pan once the oil is hot and shallow-fry for about 10 minutes. Turn the patties in around 5 minutes so that it is cooked evenly. It should be golden brown in color.

Step 4: Toast the buns lightly or use as is. Spread the tomato puree on one side of the bun and sour cream on the other side of the bun. Place the lettuce leaves, sliced tomatoes, sliced onions and the patty in between the bun. Place a toothpick in between to hold it all together and serve immediately!

CHAPTER 8

DINNER RECIPES

D inner is a time for getting together. It is a time for the family and signifies a perfect end to a long, tiring, day. At this time, a healthy meal on the dinner table can make a world of difference to rejuvenate the mood of everyone in the family. The recipes in this book are and interesting combination of world cuisine to suit a wide variety of palate. A large amount of lunch recipes given above are versatile enough to be used for dinner and vice versa. Ideally, dinner should be considerably lighter than the breakfast and lunch to promote weight loss. You will see that most of these recipes are lower in calories than the breakfast ones, yet as filling and delicious. Choosing any one of these recipes will end your day on the right note.

Healthy Quinoa Entrée

Quinoa is a lifesaver for those of us on a whole food diet. It's a flavorful, grain-like ingredient that is unbelievably rich in nutrients. To add to its glowing list of benefits, it is also low-calorie and gluten-free which makes it perfect for weight loss. This entrée combines it with sweet potatoes which by itself are much lower in calories than regular potatoes making it a tasty, delicious evening meal for those who are looking to control their weight.

Preparation Time: 10 mins

Cooking Time: 45 mins

Portions: 6

Ingredients:

3 medium sweet potatoes, peeled and chopped

1 chopped Red Onion

10 Garlic Cloves, chopped

1 tbsp of Olive Oil

1 cup Quinoa Grain

2 cups of chickpeas, soaked overnight and boiled

2 tbsp chopped green onions

Salt and Freshly Ground Black Pepper to taste

Step 1: Take a large baking dish and put the potatoes, garlic, onions, and olive oil and mix thoroughly. Spread the ingredients in the baking dish.

Step 2: Preheat the oven to about 425 degrees and put the baking dish in for around 45 mins. Stir the potatoes every 15 mins so that it is evenly cooked.

Step 3: Meanwhile, boil around 2-3 cups of water in a large pot. Once the water is warmed up, add the quinoa to it and cook on medium heat for about 10 mins. The quinoa should have absorbed the water by then and be fully cooked. Drain and keep aside.

Step 4: Take the roasted vegetables out of the oven. Mix the quinoa, chickpeas and roasted veggies in a large bowl. Add salt and pepper according to taste.

Step 5: Garnish with the chopped spring onions.

Stuffed Bell Peppers

Everyone likes to come home to a colorful dinner table. This recipe can be modified using red, yellow and green peppers and is a great dish to serve during parties. It is easy to pick up and eat and is so delicious that you keep reaching out for more. You can use almost any filling to stuff in these bell peppers but I have used a low-calorie Mexican-inspired rice for those on a whole food diet.

Preparation Time: 30 mins

Cooking Time: 15 mins

Portions: 4

Ingredients:

2 cups cooked brown rice

1 Chopped Red/White Onion

1 Chopped Green Pepper

2-3 tbsp Tomato Puree (recipe in Basics)

½ Bowl Sweet Corn

1 tsp homemade Butter

1 tbsp of olive oil

4 Uncut Bell Peppers of your choice

4-5 Minced Garlic Cloves

Salt and Pepper to taste

Step 1: Melt the butter in a large frying pan. Add the chopped garlic once the butter has heated then saute for a minute.

Step 2: Once the garlic has cooked, add the onions, chopped green peppers, sweet corn and cook them for a few minutes until they become soft. Add a pinch of salt to speed up the cooking process. Then, add the tomato puree, salt, and pepper to the vegetables. Cook for a few minutes and add the rice. Mix thoroughly so that the vegetables and the puree coat the rice completely. Remove from heat and keep aside.

Step 3: Take the whole bell peppers and slice them into halves. Remove the seeds and the white portions from inside the bell peppers. Lightly brush the bell peppers with olive oil.

Step 4: Preheat the over to around 375 degrees.

Step 5: Stuff the bell peppers with the prepared rice mixture. Place it in the oven and cook for around 15-20 mins till the peppers are cooked. Plate and serve hot.

Thai Rice Bowl

This is a great dish to add some variety to your dinner table. A burst of exotic flavors and a wholesome meal, this dish is everything that you could think of and more. Most of these ingredients are easily available at your local grocery store even if they sound unfamiliar. The great part is you can easily make this dish more palatable for older people and kids by cutting down on some of the peppers.

Preparation Time: 15 mins

Cooking Time: 30 mins

Portions: 2

Ingredients:

1 cup uncooked brown rice

1 cup homemade coconut milk

½ tbsp finely chopped ginger

½ tbsp finely chopped garlic

½ chopped green bell pepper

½ chopped red bell pepper

1 small chopped onion

2 peeled and chopped carrots

1 tbsp chopped cilantro

1 bunch chopped spring onions

2 tbsp sesame oil

½ cup roasted peanuts

1 jalapeno

Salt to taste

Step 1: To prepare the coconut milk, take a large coconut and scoop out the white portion in the center. Place the coconut chunks into a blend and blend with a little milk until it becomes a smooth puree. Drain out the excess shreds using a sieve and use the coconut milk in cooking.

Step 2: Heat around 2 cups of water in a large pot. Once the water heats up, add the rice, coconut milk, garlic, and ginger to it. Cover the pot and cook for around 30 minutes on low heat, checking it to see of the rice is cooked. Turn the heat off and keep aside once cooked. The rice should have soaked all the liquid up.

Step 3: In a separate pan, sauté all the vegetables in the sesame oil for about 5-10 minutes until fully cooked.

Step 4: Add the rice to the sautéed veggies and mix thoroughly. Transfer to a bowl to serve.

Step 5: Crush the peanuts using a grinder. Garnish the rice with the peanuts, spring onions, and the cilantro. Serve hot!

Lentil Lettuce Wrap

This dish is a perfect combination of health food and comfort food. The filling in this can be used for so many recipes. It can be had with rice, as a dip with chips or bread and anything else you can think of! The slightly Indian spices and flavors added to it make it so flavorful that it is truly a treat for your taste buds. But be warned, this dish is extremely addictive and you will frequently find yourself cooking it again and again!

Preparation Time: 15 mins

Cooking Time: 35 mins

Portions: 4-6 wraps

Ingredients:

6 Lettuce Leaves

1 cup red lentils, washed, soaked, and drained

1 red onion, chopped finely

1 tomato, chopped finely

1 red pepper, chopped finely

1 tsp chili powder

¼ tsp turmeric powder

1 tsp coriander powder

1 tsp clarified butter/ghee

2 tbsp tomato puree (recipe in basics)

Salt to taste

Step 1: Take a large pan and heat the clarified butter/ghee in it. Saute the onions, bell peppers, and chopped tomatoes until cooked for about 5 minutes.

Step 2: Add around two cups of water, lentil, and a little salt to the vegetables and let it cook on low heat for around 30 minutes. After around 10 minutes, add the chili powder, coriander powder, turmeric, and tomato puree to the pan. Mix thoroughly and let it cook while covered.

Step 3: Once the liquid is all soaked up, check if the lentils are soft. If not, add a little more water and cook for some more time. The mixture should be soft enough, so mash it thoroughly.

Step 4: Serve hot in a bowl along with washed lettuce leaves.

Whole Potato Pizza

All of us experience a pizza craving every once in a while. This healthy pizza recipe is perfect for those dinner time when we experience moments like those. Made from a tasty potato crust, you can modify it to add your favorite toppings just like you would in any other pizza. You can experiment with a pesto, tomato or a creamy sauce base. This potato crust pizza is a perfect end to any day when you want to indulge a little, but not go overboard.

Preparation Time: 30 mins

Cooking Time: 30 mins

Portions: 8 slices/ 1 pizza

Ingredients:

3 whole potatoes, boiled, peeled and mashed

2 cloves chopped garlic

¼ cup chickpea flour

¼ cup whole wheat flour

2 Tbsp Homemade yeast (recipe in Breakfast)

1 tsp dried Italian herbs

½ tsp salt

1 bowl of toppings of your choice (onions, bell peppers, mushrooms, olives)

1 bowl of cottage cheese chunks

2 tbsp fresh cream

2 tbsp tomato puree

Step 1: To prepare the sauce for the pizza, mix the tomato puree and the fresh cream and keep aside.

Step 2: Preheat the oven to around 425 degrees and grease a baking sheet with butter.

Step 3: In a large bowl, mix the mashed potatoes, flour, herbs, salt, chopped garlic and yeast. Wet you hand if needed to bind the mixture together and roll in into a round shape. Then ends will probably not be perfect because of the base. You can make the base as thick or thin as you please depending on taste.

Step 4: Transfer the base onto the baking sheet. Spread the sauce and the toppings on the base. Distribute the pieces of cottage cheese on the pizza evenly.

Step 5: Put inside the oven and bake for around 30 mins until crispy. Slice into slices using a pizza cutter and serve hot!

CHAPTER 9

Tips and Tricks

L ike any other diet, the whole food diet cannot work in isolation. It is simply an easier way to diet, where you eat and live healthy without starving yourself. This diet can have major benefits to your health if you keep in mind these simple tips and tricks.

The whole food diet has to be combined with reasonable and regular exercise in order to see definite results. A healthy lifestyle is as important as a healthy diet. Try to get in at least 5 hours of exercise a week to see immediate, weekly results.

The whole food diet does not limit you by prescribing what to eat every specific day. Diets with specific meal plans are only possible to follow for a short amount of time before they become monotonous. But, this means that you have to make your own smart choices. Make sure that you balance your meals so that if you are having a heavy, high-calorie lunch or breakfast, then balance it out with a lighter dinner or snacks.

Almost all of things that you are allowed to eat can be found at your local departmental store. Just make sure to check the labels before you buy the food. It might take a little more time but it will be much better for you in the long run!

It might be tempting to snack on junk food when the mid-day hunger pangs sneak in. Carry some chopped veggies and some homemade sour cream for a tasty, whole-food afternoon snack.

Most of the recipes in this book are easy to store for at least a week. So, if you think that preparing some of them are too time-consuming. You can easily make them during the weekend and use for the whole week!

CONCLUSION

Thank you again for downloading this book!

I hope this book was able to help you to see the benefits of the Whole Foods diet and give you a reason to follow it. With our easy 30-day Diet challenge, we are sure that you will be able to dedicate a month to healthy eating and see visible changes to your physical and mental health. You will find yourself waking up with more energy than every day and really *feel* the difference within you.

The next step is to incorporate our words into your life. If you wholeheartedly commit to the whole food diet, there is no way that you will not be able to see the difference. We hope you have a successful journey once you embark on the whole foods diet!

Finally, if you enjoyed this book, then I'd like to ask you for a favor, would you be kind enough to leave a review for this book on Amazon? It'd be greatly appreciated!

Click here to leave a review for this book on Amazon!

Thank you and good luck!

CHECK OUT MY OTHER BOOKS:

Low Carb High Fat

HCG Diet - *http://amzn.to/1KRI1V1*

Dash Diet - *http://amzn.to/1IQ2tQ5*

Medittereanean Diet - *http://amzn.to/1IXhl0F*

Anti Inflammatory Diet - *http://amzn.to/1O3NgSB*

Below you'll find some of my other popular books that are popular on Amazon and Kindle as well. Simply click on the links below to check them out. Alternatively, you can visit my author page on Amazon to see other work done by me.

If the links do not work, for whatever reason, you can simply search for these titles on the Amazon website to find them.